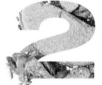
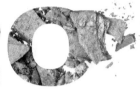

BEAUTY MYTHS
BUSTED!

What Really Works for
Clear, Younger-Looking Skin

Paula Begoun

& THE PAULA'S CHOICE RESEARCH TEAM

D1374312

Copyright © 2013, Paula Begoun
Publisher: Paula's Choice, LLC.
705 5th Avenue South, Suite 200
Seattle, Washington 98104

First Edition Printing: April 2013

ISBN: 978-1-877988-36-3
10 9 8 7 6 5 4 3 2 1

PAULA'S CHOICE
——— SKINCARE ———

Dedicated to **helping you find the best products** for your skin
...whether you use our products or someone else's!

In a world where we are constantly bombarded with misleading information from the cosmetics industry, Paula's Choice is a truly unique company. Our goal is to help you find the best products for your skin, whether you use Paula's Choice products or products from other brands. Since 1979, internationally known Cosmetics Cop Paula Begoun and her research team have worked tirelessly to cut through the hype, revealing the truth behind beauty myths that waste your money or hurt your skin. We base our recommendations only on published scientific research, not on what fashion magazines state or company-sponsored research shows.

At *Beautypedia.com*, we review thousands of beauty products so you can find the best products and avoid the worst—because wasting money and harming your skin isn't pretty.

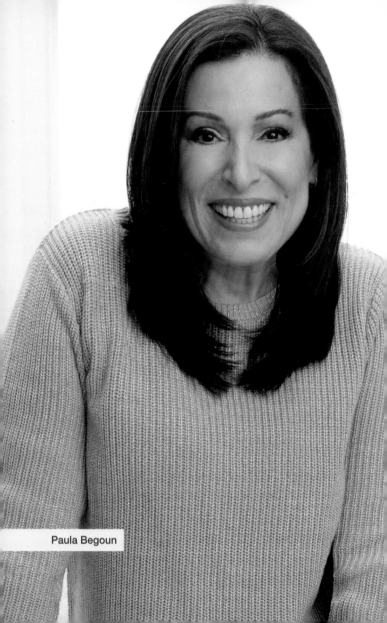
Paula Begoun

PAULA'S STORY

"At the age of 11 I began a tormented struggle with acne. I tried numerous skin-care products and medical treatments—yet my skin didn't get any better. Then, more than a decade later at the age of 25 (I'll never forget this moment), **I read the ingredient label on a skin-care product I was using and the fourth ingredient was acetone. That's nail polish remover! No wonder my skin wasn't getting better.** From that moment on, I read all of the research I could find on skin care. Eventually I was able to put together a skin-care routine that completely transformed my skin.

After suffering all those years, I wanted to do everything possible to prevent others from going through the same pain. So I started writing books and doing TV appearances to tell the world which skin-care products really work—and which are a waste of money or actually make skin worse. Together with my talented team, I've written 20 books, including the current edition of my product review guide, ***Don't Go to the Cosmetics Counter Without Me***. In print and online at *Beautypedia.com*, we review more than 45,000 skin-care and makeup products so that everyone can know which products are best for their skin type and concerns.

In 1995, I decided to put my years of research on skin-care ingredients to use, and created the Paula's Choice line of products. My team and I make sure these products contain only ingredients that are proven by science to correct skin concerns, including acne and wrinkles. **Each product is clinically proven to be non-irritating, 100% fragrance-free, dye-free, and never tested on animals.**"

Thank you,

Paula Begoun

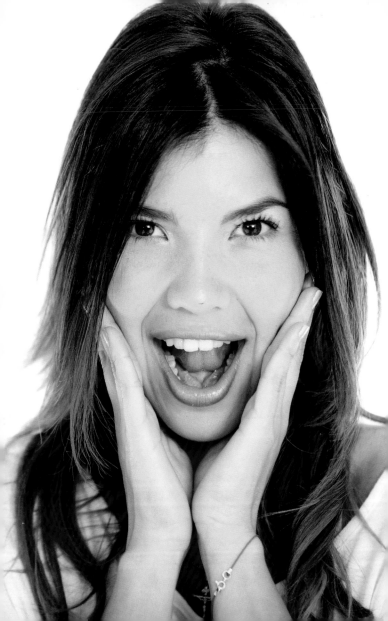

THE **20** MOST **SHOCKING**
Beauty Myths and the Real Facts!

What consumers are led to believe about skin care and makeup could fill volumes. There's so much information that getting to the truth is almost impossible, so we're here to tell you what's really possible—and what's worth your time and money based on published research, not on marketing spin or fabrications.

The myths that follow are only a snapshot of the typical erroneous information you get from cosmetics companies or so-called skin-care "experts"— information that ends up hurting your skin and your budget. For more facts on skin care, makeup, and hair care, please visit us at *Beautypedia.com*!

MYTH #1:

When shopping for skin-care products, age is an important factor, especially if you have "mature skin."

Many products on the market claim to be designed for a specific age group, especially for "mature" women. "Mature" usually refers to women over 50. However, everyone between the ages of 50 and 100 does not have the same skin-care needs.

What you need to know is that age is not a skin type; that is, not everyone in the same age group has the same skin type—and **choosing products based on your age is not a wise way to shop**. Your skin-care routine should depend strictly on your skin type and concerns. **No matter your age, if your skin is oily, you should not be using the same products as someone with dry skin**.

How dry, sun-damaged, oily, sensitive, thin, blemished, or normal your skin is has nothing to do with your age. And then, there are the issues of skin conditions such as rosacea, psoriasis, allergies, and other skin disorders, which again, have nothing to do with age.

Turning 50 does not mean a woman should assume her skin is drying up and, therefore, that she must begin using "mature" skin-care products, which, almost always, are products designed for dry skin that are no different from any of the other skin-care products for dry skin on the market.

For many women over 50 (including Paula), it definitely does not mean that the battle with blemishes is over. Women of any age can also struggle with sensitive skin.

To find the best products for your skin type and to learn more about taking the best care of your skin, visit us at *Beautypedia.com*.

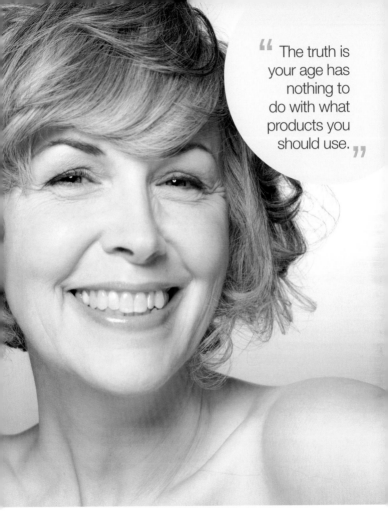

" The truth is your age has nothing to do with what products you should use. "

Sources: *British Journal of Community Nursing, May 2007, pages 203–204; Journal of Investigative Dermatology, December 2005, pages 364–368; Journal of Vascular Surgery, October 1999, pages 734–743; International Journal of Cosmetic Science, October 2007, pages 409–410; and Cutaneous and Ocular Toxicology, April 2007, pages 343–357.*

MYTH #2:

Hypoallergenic, dermatologist-tested, and cosmeceutical products are better for skin than other products.

"Hypoallergenic" is nothing more than an advertising contrivance meant to imply that a product is unlikely or less likely to cause allergic reactions and, therefore, is better for sensitive or problem skin.

The truth? There are absolutely no accepted testing methods, ingredient restrictions, regulations, guidelines, rules, or procedures of any kind, anywhere in the world, for determining whether or not a product qualifies as being "hypoallergenic." A company can label any product they sell as "hypoallergenic" because there is no regulation that says they can't, regardless of any supposed "proof" they may claim to have. Really, what proof can they provide given that there is no standard against which to measure?

It is quite surprising how many products that claim to be "hypoallergenic" actually contain problematic ingredients that can indeed trigger allergic or sensitizing skin reactions. Unfortunately, the word "hypoallergenic" gives you no better understanding of what you are, or aren't, putting on your skin.

The terms "dermatologist-tested" and "cosmeceutical" are also incredibly misleading. "Dermatologist-tested" is nothing more than a marketing gimmick; the companies know that people believe doctors have the consumer's best interest at heart or assume that they know more about skin care—but that is often not the case. We've reviewed lots of products endorsed by dermatologists that are either not worth the money or are poorly formulated.

The primary problem with the term "dermatologist-tested" is that often it does not tell you which dermatologist did the testing; what he or she tested; how he or she performed the testing; or what the results were. Plus, the company has almost always hired the dermatologist who does the testing (there are lots of doctors on the payroll of lots of cosmetics companies).

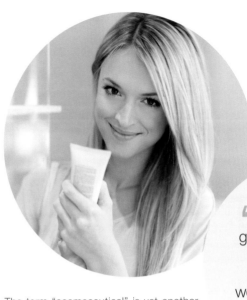

"Advertising gimmicks and misleading information won't help you take care of your skin."

The term "cosmeceutical" is yet another advertising gimmick created by cosmetics companies and dermatologists to suggest that their "cosmeceutical" products are somehow better than other products in the cosmetics industry. When you hear the word "cosmeceutical," you're supposed to think a product contains pharmaceutical-grade ingredients and, therefore, it must be better for your skin, right?

The fact is, "cosmeceutical" has no legal, regulated, or recognized meaning as to what distinguishes it from non-cosmeceutical. A quick comparison of ingredient lists reveals that there is nothing any more unique or medical about cosmeceuticals than any other skin-care product. Plus, the term isn't regulated, so any cosmetics company can use it, regardless of what their products contain.

Sources: www.fda.gov; and Ostomy and Wound Management, March 2003, pages 20–21.

MYTH #3:

There are skin-care products that can work like Botox or dermal fillers.

There is absolutely no research showing that any skin-care product can work—even remotely—in any manner like Botox or dermal fillers (such as Restylane or Aretcoll) or laser resurfacing (such as Fraxel). Regardless of the ingredients or the claims for skin-care products, it just isn't possible. Even Botox can't work like Botox if you apply it topically rather than injecting it into facial muscles. Nor can dermal fillers plump up wrinkles when applied topically rather than injected.

When administered by professionals, Botox and dermal fillers almost immediately make wrinkles in the treated area disappear. Believing that a skin-care product can do the same thing, over any length of time, is a complete waste of money. There has never been a single skin-care product that has ever put a plastic surgeon or cosmetic dermatologist out of business!

If skin-care products did work like Botox or dermal fillers, they would be exceedingly dangerous to use. Just think, if a product did work like Botox to "relax" or paralyze muscles, you wouldn't want that all over your face because it could lead to drooping and sagging skin. And how would you be able to control the application? And, if a product did work like dermal fillers, it would plump up skin all over and you would have a bloated face because, again, there is no way to control application. Thankfully, that cannot happen!

Sources: *Journal of Neural Transmission, April 2008, pages 617–623; Laryngoscope, May 2008, pages 790–796; Expert Opinion on Pharmacotherapy, June 2007, pages 1059–1072; Journal of Headache and Pain, October 2007, pages 294–300; Pediatrics, July 2007, pages 49–58; Clinical and Plastic Surgery, April 2005, pages 151–162; Plastic and Reconstructive Surgery, November 2007, pages 33S–40S; Dermatologic Therapy, May 2006, pages 141–150; Dermatologic Surgery, June 2008, Supplemental, pages S92–S99, and December 2007, Supplemental, pages S168–S175; Plastic and Reconstructive Surgery, November 2007, Supplemental, pages S17–S26; Journal of Cosmetic Laser Therapy, December 2005, pages171–176; Dermatology, April 2006, pages 300–304; and Aesthetic and Plastic Surgery, January-February 2005, pages 34–48.*

MYTH #4:

If a company claims to have studies proving a product works, that means it does work.

It would be great if that were always true, but all of us must admit, from experience, that it isn't.

In the world of skin care, there is an entire business known as claim substantiation and it does not always equate to legitimate scientific research at all. Here's how it works:

Laboratories, including labs at some universities and colleges, set up a study so that the results support whatever the label or advertisements say that a product can do. Once these so-called studies are complete, many cosmetics companies publish their results in quasi-medical journals like *Cosmetic Dermatology* or post them on their websites.

They can seem very convincing, but **there are lots of ways to use pseudo-science to create "proof" for a claim that, in reality, has very little to do with science and everything to do with marketing.**

Something else to consider is the fact that the new products companies launch often have the same claims, with the same kinds of so-called studies supporting those claims. If the studies show the same results, then why launch new products? And, more often than not, the new products cost a lot more than the previous "miracle" product they're replacing.

Sources: *Cosmetic Claims Substantiation, Cosmetic Science and Technology Series, vol. 18, ed. Louise Aust, New York: Marcel Dekker, 1998; and Cosmetics and Toiletries, article: "The European Group on Efficacy Measurement of Cosmetics and Other Topical Products is considering new cosmetic legislation to regulate claims of efficacy," Pierard, G. E. Masson, Ph., Allured Publishing Corp, 2000.*

"The reality is no skin-care product exists that works like Botox or any other medical procedure."

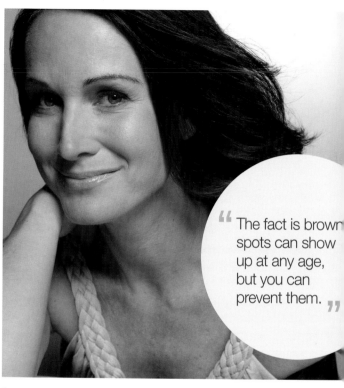

“ The fact is brown spots can show up at any age, but you can prevent them. ”

Sources: Journal of Cosmetic Dermatology, September 2007, pages 195–202; Dermatology Nursing, October 2004, pages 401–413; Age and Ageing, March 2006, pages 110–115; Journal of Cutaneous Medicine and Surgery, May-June 2008, pages 107–113; Journal of Investigative Dermatology Symposium Proceedings, April 2008, pages 20–24; Experimental Dermatology, August 2005, pages 601–608; Bioscience, Biotechnology, and Biochemistry, December 2005, pages 2368–2373; International Journal of Dermatology, August 2004, pages 604–607; Journal of Drugs in Dermatology, July-August 2004, pages 377–381; Facial and Plastic Surgery, February 2004, pages 3–9; Dermatologic Surgery, March 2004, pages 385–388; Journal of Bioscience and Bioengineering, March 2005, pages 272–276; The Lancet, August 2007, pages 528–537; Skin Pharmacology and Physiology, June 2005, pages 253–262; and Journal of the American Academy of Dermatology, December 2006, pages 1048–1065.

MYTH #5:
Dark brown discolorations are caused by age.

First, the term "age spot" is really a misnomer. **Brown, freckle-like skin discolorations are not a result of age; they are the result of years of unprotected sun exposure.** They really should be called sun spots or sun-induced discolorations because exposure to sunlight is what causes them, and knowing that will help you be better able to get rid of them and prevent them from occurring in the first place.

Sun spots can show up at any age, and treating sun-induced brown discolorations doesn't necessarily require a specialty product. It does require, however, proven ingredients such as hydroquinone, niacinamide, forms of vitamin C, and select plant extracts (detailed below), and diligent daily application of sunscreen to make a noticeable, lasting difference.

And, be sure not to forget the backs of your hands and your chest. For hands, you must reapply every time you wash them because sunscreen does wash off. We know it's a pain to do this, but we promise you will love the results!

For treating discolorations, the ingredient hydroquinone has the highest efficacy for lightening skin and a long history of safe use behind it. There are alternatives (mostly plant extracts) that show promise for lightening skin, but there isn't as much research supporting their efficacy and they don't work as well as hydroquinone.

Other promising skin-lightening ingredients include licorice extract (specifically glabridin), azelaic acid, arbutin and its derivatives, stabilized vitamin C (L-ascorbic acid, ascorbic acid, and magnesium ascorbyl phosphate), flavonoids, hesperidin, niacinamide, and polyphenols. These may be used as a blend with or without hydroquinone. By the way, you can read more about these and other ingredients by visiting the Cosmetic Ingredient Dictionary section of our ***Beautypedia.com*** website! You can find the best skin lightening products on this site as well.

MYTH #6:
You'll eventually outgrow acne.

> " The truth is women between the ages of 12 and 65 can have acne! "

Women in their 20s, 30s, 40s, 50s, and 60s can have acne, just like teenagers, and the treatment options are the same regardless of age. Not everyone who has acne as a teenager will grow out of it and even if you had clear skin as a teenager, there's no guarantee that you won't suffer from acne later in life, perhaps during menopause. You can blame this often-maddening inconsistency on hormones!

It is true that men can outgrow acne, because after puberty men's hormone levels even out, while women's hormone levels fluctuate throughout their lifetime, which is why many women experience breakouts around their menstrual cycle.

To find the best rated products for controlling acne and blemishes, visit us at *Beautypedia.com*.

Sources: British Journal of Dermatology, December 2012, ePublication; Indian Journal of Dermatology, Venereology, and Leprology, May-June 2012, pages 335–341; and Journal of Women's Health, February 2012, pages 223–230.

DID YOU KNOW?

Treating acne remains the same whether you're a teen or an adult. "Adult acne" doesn't require special products, though you may find breakouts during adulthood to be less frequent yet more severe. Even so, the core treatment options remain the same: Gentle cleansing, killing acne-causing bacteria with benzoyl peroxide, and exfoliating with salicylic acid (also know as beta hydroxy acid or BHA).

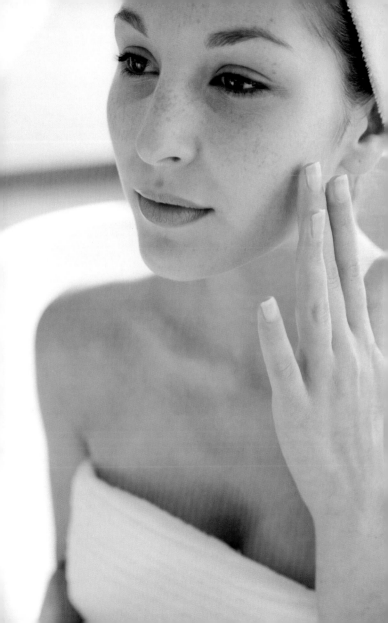

MYTH #7:
Makeup causes acne.

There is no research indicating that makeup of any kind causes acne, and there is no consensus on which ingredients or combinations of ingredients are problematic. Makeup in stick form may be more likely to cause breakouts, but that's true of skin-care products in stick form, too, and even then, despite what you may have read on blogs or beauty forums, there are no absolutes.

In the late 1970s, there was some research performed on rabbit skin using 100% concentrations of ingredients to determine whether or not they caused acne, but very few makeup products use 100% of any one ingredient. Consequently, it was determined that this study had nothing to do with the way women wear makeup (or use skin-care products for that matter), and it was never repeated or considered helpful.

Still, women do experience breakouts after using makeup, especially if they sleep in their makeup. Sleeping in makeup can be irritating to skin and that can cause breakouts, plus it means you aren't removing built-up dead skin cells and debris that can clog pores.

To find the best products to reduce or prevent breakouts, visit us at *Beautypedia.com*.

The terms "noncomedogenic" and "non-acnegenic" are meaningless. The cosmetics industry uses these claims to indicate that a product is less likely to clog pores and cause breakouts, but there is no established standard or regulation anywhere in the world to go by. Any product can make this claim, regardless of what it contains.

MYTH #8:

Everyone needs an eye cream or product for the eye area.

This one may shock you, but **there is no evidence, research, or documentation validating the claim that the eye area needs skin-care ingredients that are different from those you use on your face** (or neck area or décolletage) when it comes to fighting wrinkles, skin discolorations, or sagging or dry skin.

> " You should never apply products containing irritating ingredients, period! "

Even if there were ingredients that were special for the eye area but useless for the rest of the face, that certainly isn't evident in products sold specifically for the eye area. In fact, their formulations are random, with no consistency whatsoever. All cosmetics companies put whatever ingredients they want into their eye products. Read the ingredient labels on these "specialty" products. They will more than prove our point.

Occasionally, a physician, aesthetician, or someone selling skin-care products will defend their eye creams by telling us that the eye area doesn't need ingredients that cause irritation. We agree wholeheartedly with that statement, but the same is absolutely true for skin on your face or anywhere else on your body! You shouldn't be applying formulations with irritating ingredients, period! **All your eye area needs is a well-formulated product, and that can certainly be the same product you use on your face, or, if you prefer, a well-formulated eye cream.**

What if the skin around your eyes is drier than the rest of your face? That's fairly common, but it still doesn't mean everyone needs an eye cream. You can treat your eye area with a more emollient, fragrance-free facial moisturizer or, if you prefer, an eye cream. A well-formulated facial serum is another great option to use around the eyes. The bottom line: Not everyone needs an eye cream, but if you prefer to use one, make sure it's a great formula.

MYTH #9:
There's a product out there that erases wrinkles.

Regrettably, there is no magic potion or combination of products in any price range that can make wrinkles truly disappear. **There are things you can do to make a huge difference in their appearance, but "erasing" and the other over-the-top claims you've seen for antiwrinkle products just aren't true.**

Most of the wrinkles you see are the result of cumulative sun damage and the inevitable breakdown of your skin's natural support structure. Skin-care ingredients, no matter who is selling them or what claims they make for them, cannot replace what plastic surgeons and cosmetic dermatologists can do. There are literally thousands of antiwrinkle products being sold, and we buy more of these than almost any other beauty product. But despite this onslaught of products, plastic surgeons and cosmetic dermatologists are not going out of business.

What are the skin-care-related things you can do to reduce wrinkles and prevent them from occurring? Regular use of brilliantly formulated sunscreens, exfoliants (AHAs or BHA), moisturizers loaded with antioxidants and cell-communicating ingredients, and retinoids (components of Vitamin A including retinol), among numerous others are your best options, and this is supported by copious research.

The take away from this that will save you thousands of dollars is that most antiwrinkle and anti-aging skin-care products don't perform as the exaggerated claims on the label would lead you to believe—and that remains true, product launch after product launch.

MYTH #10:

Expensive cosmetics are better than inexpensive ones.

The absolute truth is that there are good and bad products in all price categories. It's all about the formulation, not the price.

The amount of money you spend on skin-care products has nothing to do with the quality or uniqueness of the formula. You would be shocked at how many expensive products are little more than water and wax and at how many inexpensive products are beautifully formulated and outright beauty bargains.

Spending less doesn't hurt your skin, and spending more doesn't help it. Again, it's all about the formulation, not the price. Besides, haven't most of us splurged on products that we assumed would be better due to their cost, and found that they were big disappointments? Visit *Beautypedia.com* to see thousands of unbiased reviews based on published research, not marketing hype.

DOLLARS&SENSE

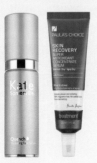

KATE SOMERVILLE
Quench Hydrating
Face Serum

$75
(1 oz.)

PAULA'S CHOICE
Skin Recovery
Super Antioxidant
Concentrate Serum

$30
(1 oz.)

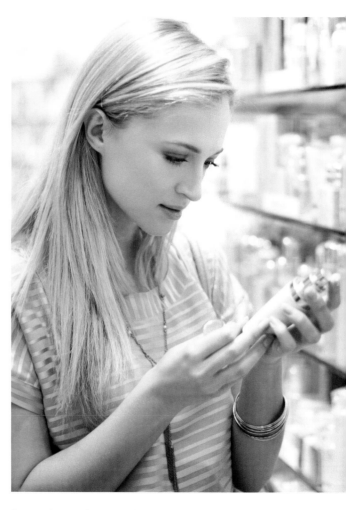

Sources: *Journal of Dermatologic Science, May 2008, pages 135–142; International Journal of Cosmetic Science, October 2007, pages 385–390; Dermatitis, September 2004, pages 109–116; and International Wound Journal, September 2006, pages 181–187.*

MYTH #11:
Mineral oil and petrolatum are the worst skin-care ingredients around.

Poor mineral oil and petrolatum—always being picked on! Simply put, everything bad you've heard or read about these ingredients is not accurate. Although mineral oil does originate from crude oil (petroleum), it is as natural as any other earth-derived substance, including plants and minerals. Moreover, lots of ingredients are derived from awful-sounding sources but are, nevertheless, benign and totally safe. **According to research, mineral oil and petrolatum are not only safe for skin, but are also great ingredients for healing dry skin!**

Cosmetics-grade mineral oil and petrolatum are among the most nonirritating moisturizing ingredients available. Yes, they can reduce the amount of air that comes in contact with skin, but that's what a good antioxidant is supposed to do; they don't suffocate skin! No one has ever had necrotic (dead) skin from applying mineral oil or petrolatum, especially babies! **In fact, there are several studies showing that pure mineral oil helps heal and moisturize skin quite effectively.**

The mineral oil in skin-care products is certified as either USP (United States Pharmacopeia) or BP (British Pharmacopeia), and it's completely safe, soothing, and healthy for skin. It does not contain impurities that harm skin in any way.

In terms of impurities falsely associated with cosmetics-grade mineral oil and petrolatum, you may be surprised to learn that plants are subject to impurities, too. Plants come out of the ground, with insects, worms, mold, fungus, bacteria, and other impurities that must be cleaned (or cut) off before they can be put into a cosmetic, just like mineral oil and petrolatum.

By the way, despite their greasy feel, neither mineral oil nor petrolatum can clog pores. Both remain on the surface of skin, where they do the most good, although those with oily skin may not like how they feel or look on skin.

MYTH #12:
Natural ingredients are better for skin than synthetic ingredients.

There is no factual basis or scientific legitimacy for that belief. It's an emotional belief, not one based on logic.

Not only is the definition of "natural" hazy, but the term is loosely regulated, so any cosmetics company can use it to mean whatever they want it to mean. Plus, **just because an ingredient grows out of the ground or is found in nature doesn't make it automatically good for skin. The reverse is also true: Just because it is synthetic doesn't make it bad for skin.**

"Consumers should not necessarily assume that an 'organic' or 'natural' ingredient or product would possess greater inherent safety than another chemically identical version of the same ingredient," said Dr. Linda M. Katz, director of the Food and Drug Administration's Office of Cosmetics and Colors (New York Times, November 1, 2007). **"In fact, 'natural' ingredients may be harder to preserve against microbial contamination and growth than synthetic raw materials."**

"But people should not interpret even the USDA Organic seal or any organic seal of approval on cosmetics as proof of health benefits or of efficacy," said Joan Shaffer, USDA spokeswoman. The National Organic Program is a marketing program, not a safety program. Steak may be graded prime by the USDA, but that has no bearing on whether it is safe or nutritious to eat.

Ideally, the skin-care products you choose should contain a mix of beneficial ingredients, both natural and synthetic. When properly formulated, these ingredients work in harmony to give your skin the best that natural and synthetic have to offer, and you'll see the difference. If you prefer to use products with mostly or all natural ingredients, visit us at *Beautypedia.com*, where we review many products claiming to be natural. You'll quickly find out which ones are the best to use.

Source: www.ams.usda.gov/nop/FactSheets/Backgrounder.html.

MYTH #13:

Products that make skin feel cool or tingly are good.

heck out
e Ingredient
ctionary at
eautypedia.com
r details on
ousands
ingredients! „

Fact: A cooling or tingling sensation is your skin telling you it is being irritated, nothing more. That familiar tingling sensation is your skin responding to irritation, resulting in inflammation. **Products that produce this sensation can damage your skin's healing process,** make scarring worse, cause collagen and elastin to break down, and increase the growth of bacteria that cause acne.

Ingredients that cause a cooling or tingling sensation are considered counter-irritants. Counter-irritants cause local inflammation in an effort to reduce inflammation in deeper or adjacent tissues, such as to relieve pain in muscles or joints. In other words, they substitute one kind of inflammation for another, but inflammation is never good for the skin. Ingredients such as menthol, menthyl lactate, peppermint, camphor, and other types of mint are counter-irritants and they show up in many skin (and lip) products.

Irritation impairs the skin's immune and healing response. And, **although your skin may not show it or may not react in an irritated fashion, if you apply irritants to your skin the damage is still taking place**—it's just that it's taking place below the skin's surface—and it is ongoing and adds up over time. Much like you don't feel the damage that is occurring from unprotected sun exposure during the day, you often don't feel the negative effect of irritating ingredients on the skin—but, left unprotected, you'll eventually see the damage.

Sources: Skin Research and Technology, November 2001, pages 227–237; Skin Pharmacology and Applied Skin Physiology, November-December 2000, pages 358–371; Archives of Dermatologic Research, May 1996, pages 245–248; Code of Federal Regulations Title 21-Food and Drugs, revised April 1, 2001, CITE: 21CFR310.545, www.fda.gov; and www. naturaldatabase.com.

MYTH #14:
Blackheads can be washed or scrubbed away.

Blackheads may make skin look dirty, but they are not related to dirt or to how often you wash or scrub your face. (As a general rule, scrubbing skin is never a wise move.)

Blackheads develop when a clog forms within the pore and prevents oil and cellular debris from exiting the pore normally. Clogs can form for a couple of reasons. One, hormones cause too much sebum (oil) to be produced inside the pore, which causes dead skin cells to accumulate and get in the way. Two, the pore itself is impaired or misshapen such that the pathway for the oil to exit through the pore is blocked, creating a clog. As the clog nears the surface of the skin, the mixture of oil and cellular debris oxidizes and turns—you guessed it—black.

You cannot scrub away blackheads, at least not completely. Using a topical scrub can remove the top portion of the blackhead, but it does nothing to address the underlying cause, so they're back again before too long. Think of it like pulling a weed without reaching its roots—in almost no time, the weed is back, annoying as ever.

" Salicylic ac is a superst. ingredient f getting rid blackhead

Instead of just using a scrub, try using a well-formulated BHA (salicylic acid) product. **Salicylic acid (BHA) can penetrate the oil and exfoliate inside the pore, dissolving oil and the dead skin cells that lead to constant blackheads.** Visit *Beautypedia.com* to find the best-formulated BHA (salicylic acid) products for your skin type.

Manual exfoliation can definitely be helpful, but instead of using a scrub (which often contains abrasive, irritating ingredients) consider using a soft washcloth with your gentle water-soluble cleanser instead. It's not only less expensive, but also better for your skin!

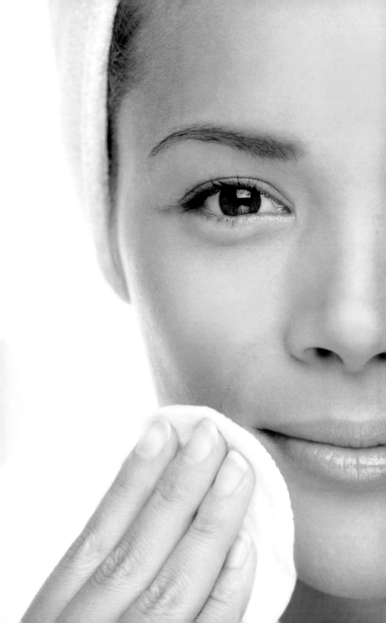

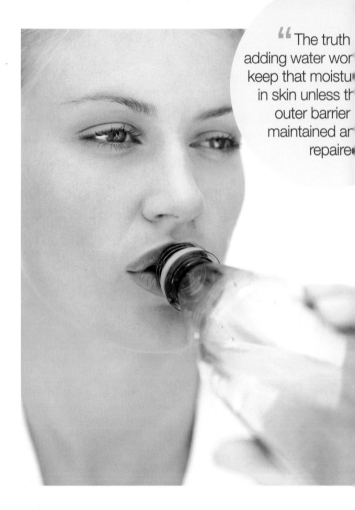

" The truth [...]
adding water wor[...]
keep that moistu[...]
in skin unless th[...]
outer barrier [...]
maintained ar[...]
repaire[...]

Sources: *British Journal of Dermatology, July 2008, pages 23–34; Dermatologic Therapy, March 2004, Supplement 1, pages 43–48; Journal of Cosmetic Dermatology, June 2007, pages 75–82; and International Journal of Cosmetic Science, April 2003, pages 63–95, and October 2000, pages 371–383.*

MYTH #15:
Dry skin? Drink more water!

If only this tip were true, it would be so easy to never have dry skin again! Ironically, dry skin is not as simple as just a lack of moisture. **Drinking more water won't make dry skin look or feel better because the water you drink does not move to the surface layers of skin, where dry skin occurs.**

You may be shocked to learn that water itself is not a good moisturizer for skin. Studies that have compared the water content of dry skin with that of normal or oily skin show that there is no statistically significant difference. Plus, adding more moisture to the skin is not necessarily a good thing. If anything, too much moisture, like soaking in a bathtub, is bad for skin because it disrupts the skin's outer barrier (the intracellular matrix) by breaking down the substances that keep skin cells functioning normally and in good shape.

It is thought that dry skin occurs when the substances between skin cells that keep them intact and smooth and healthy become depleted or damaged, bringing about a rough, uneven, and flaky texture that allows water loss. But here's the kicker: Adding water won't keep that moisture in skin unless the outer barrier is maintained or repaired.

To prevent dry skin, the primary goal is to avoid and reduce anything that damages the outer barrier, including sun damage, products that contain irritating ingredients, alcohol, drying cleansers, and smoking. All of the research about dry skin is related to the ingredients and treatments that reinforce the substances in skin that keep it functioning normally. Examples of such ingredients are glycerin, hyaluronic acid, cholesterol, ceramides, and phospholipids.

So, drinking water is all well and good, but that won't change or prevent dry skin in any way. When you drink more water than your body needs, it just means you'll be running to the bathroom more often. **The causes of and treatments for dry skin are far more complicated than water consumption.**

MYTH #16:

You can stop oily skin with the right products.

While you can definitely make skin look less oily by absorbing excess surface oil, it is almost impossible to stop skin from producing oil by using skin-care products.

Oil production is triggered by hormones within the body, primarily male hormones called androgens, which are present in both men and women. The female hormone estrogen also plays a role, but to a lesser extent.

You can't stop these hormones from being produced by applying skin-care products. You can, however, reduce the amount of androgens that are present directly inside the pore that stimulate some of the oil production. It turns out that the sebaceous (oil) gland itself also produces active androgens, which can increase sebum (oil) production.

What can happen is that stress-sensing nerves in skin respond to inflammation and irritation at the base of the pore where the oil gland resides, triggering the release of androgens. The result? The production of more oil, which can clog and enlarge pores! **It's essential to stop using skin-care products that contain irritating ingredients. Although this does not affect the production of hormones inside the body, it can make a vast improvement in how oily your skin is.**

Also helpful is to use a product containing forms of vitamin A (also called retinoids), such as retinol or prescription tretinoin, to improve the shape of the pore, which allows the oil to flow more evenly and helps prevent clogging. There is some research that niacinamide in skin-care products can also make a significant improvement.

Another thing you can do to avoid making matters worse is to not use products that contain thick, emollient ingredients. These just add to the amount of "grease" on your skin. **It also helps to absorb surface oil by using powders, mattifiers, or clay masks, but avoid masks that contain irritating ingredients.** For the best products to accomplish all this and provide long-lasting results, visit us at *Beautypedia.com*!

Sources: Experimental Dermatology, June 2008, pages 542–551; and Clinical Dermatology, September-October 2004, pages 360–366.

MYTH #17:
Moisturizer applied at night must be labeled "night cream."

The ONLY difference between a daytime and nighttime moisturizer should be that the daytime version must offer exceptional sun protection with a rating of SPF 15 or greater (and greater is better).

What you often hear from lots of sources, including misinformed physicians, is that the skin needs different ingredients at night than during the day. They usually state that skin does more repair work at night, so it needs more repairing ingredients to assist in this nightly renewal process. However, there is not a shred of research that supports this, nor is there a list anywhere of what those nighttime ingredients should be.

In reality, skin continually repairs itself and produces new skin cells, all the time, day and night. Helping skin do that in as healthy a manner as possible doesn't change based on the time of day or night. Research shows that the same beneficial ingredients work, both day and night.

At any time, skin needs a generous amount of antioxidants, cell-communicating ingredients, and skin-identical (repairing) ingredients. Using these ingredients only at nighttime is cheating your skin of the benefits it could be gaining during the daylight hours, too!

MYTH #18:
Your skin adapts to products so they eventually stop working.

Skin does not adapt to skin-care products, not any more than your body adapts to a healthy diet. Spinach and berries are healthy for you and they continue to be healthy for you, even if you eat them every day from birth to death. The same is true for your skin: As long as you are applying what is healthy for skin (and avoiding negative external sources such as unprotected sun exposure), it remains healthy.

You may note that your skin stops showing the dramatic improvement it showed initially when you first started using a specific product or routine, but that stands to reason: If you were using products with irritating or drying ingredients and then you switch to brilliantly formulated products, the initial improvement you see is going to be much more dramatic than what you'll see months later, when your skin is merely maintaining its new-found healthy, younger appearance. Again, the diet analogy applies: If you go from eating poorly to eating healthy, the initial changes will be much more dramatic than any changes you'll see and feel months down the road.

MYTH #19:
You should just use the products you like, no matter what they contain.

Lots of people have problems with their skin because they often like what isn't good for their skin. But, once you know something isn't helpful for skin, it's much harder to justify it to yourself to keep using it.

For example, you may like the day cream you're using, but if it doesn't contain sunscreen it leaves your skin wide open to sun damage. Or, you may like a moisturizer that's packaged in a jar, but most state-of-the-art ingredients,

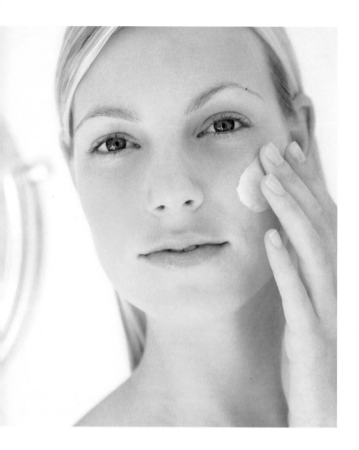

especially antioxidants, plant extracts, vitamins, and cell-communicating ingredients such as retinol, deteriorate quickly in the presence of air.

This doesn't mean that you shouldn't use products you like, but you must choose those products from among the ones that are truly healthy and beneficial for skin. To find the best products for your skin, visit us at *Beautypedia.com.*

MYTH #20:
Packaging doesn't matter when it comes to skin-care products.

Packaging plays a significant role in the stability and effectiveness of the products you use. Many state-of-the-art ingredients, from cell-communicating ingredients to antioxidants to plant extracts to skin-identical ingredients, lose their effectiveness in the presence of air. Jar packaging, once opened, permits air to enter freely, which causes these important ingredients (the very ingredients that make a product most beneficial for skin) to break down and deteriorate.

Jars also mean you are sticking your fingers into the product with each use, transferring bacteria into the product, which causes the great ingredients to break down further. Think about how long an unprotected head of lettuce lasts in your refrigerator or how long, after opening a can or jar of food, it takes for it to become a moldy mess?

Airtight packaging, or any packaging that reduces a product's exposure to air, is essential when you are buying the best products for your skin. You should also avoid clear packaging that lets light into the product. Light of any kind is a problem because it causes sensitive ingredients (like retinol) to break down.

Sources: Free Radical Biology and Medicine, September 2007, pages 818–829; Ageing Research Reviews, December 2007, pages 271–288; Dermatologic Therapy, September-October 2007, pages 314–321; International Journal of Pharmaceutics, June 12, 2005, pages 197–203; Pharmaceutical Development and Technology, January 2002, pages 1–32; International Society for Horticultural Science, www.actahort.org/members/showpdf?booknrarnr=778_5; and www.beautypackaging.com/articles/2007/03/airless-packaging.php.

BONUS MYTH!
Damaged hair can be repaired.

100% false! How many hair-care products have you bought that said they would repair or "reconstruct" damaged hair, only to have your hair return to the original state of affairs after the next washing or when the weather changed? Products such as conditioners, styling creams, gels, and shine serums can help make hair feel (and to some extent look) repaired, but once the damage is done, there's no going back. **The only surefire way to "repair" damaged hair is to cut off the damaged portion. Beyond that, the key is to minimize the damage to your hair by handling it gently and as infrequently as possible.**

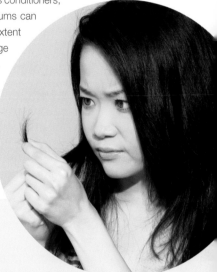

FAST HAIR FACTS:

- Hair is dead and cannot be repaired once damaged.
- There are no shampoos that can help color-treated hair last longer.
- The two biggest causes of fading hair color are water and sunlight.
- The less you touch, brush, or otherwise manipulate hair, the healthier it will be.
- No product can completely protect hair from heat damage, so ignore that claim.

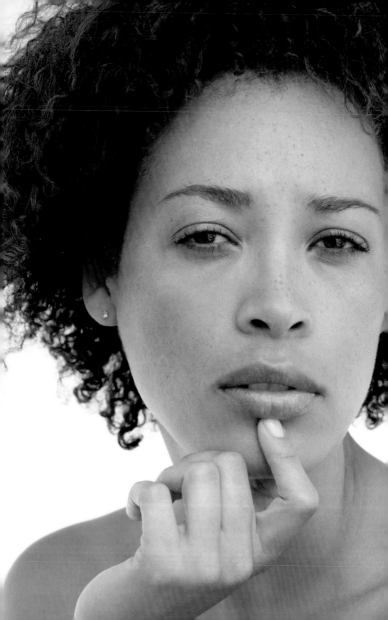

YOUR **MOST** COMMON
Skin-Care Questions
ANSWERED

What's the difference between AHA and BHA exfoliants? Do I need both?

When properly formulated, both AHAs (typically glycolic or lactic acid) and BHA (salicylic acid) are brilliant options for exfoliating the surface of skin. Both are anti-aging in that they work to reduce wrinkles, stimulate collagen, and firm the skin, but each has special qualities you'll want to consider when deciding which one to use:

- **AHAs are preferred for sun-damaged and dry skin** because they exfoliate on the surface of skin and have the added benefit of improving the skin's moisture content.

- **BHA is preferred for oily, acne-prone skin and for treating blackheads and white bumps** because BHA can get through the oil that's clogging your pores and normalize the lining of the misshapen pore that contributes to breakouts.

- **BHA has anti-inflammatory and antibacterial action**, two more reasons to use a BHA exfoliant if you have acne or sensitive, reddened skin (including rosacea).

If your skin is sun-damaged and you're also struggling with acne or clogged pores, add a BHA product to your routine.

If you'd like to use an AHA and BHA at the same time, that is an option, although not really necessary. Some people find they work well when they're applied at the same time, but if you want to give this a try, it is best to apply them separately, one during the day and one in the evening.

There are so many products in my routine. Do I really have to use all of them day and night?

We know a complete skin-care routine can seem complicated, but more often than not it can mean the difference between having the skin you want or not. It is truly helpful to follow a consistent routine, but it is also okay to skip some steps. **Start with just a simple routine and then gradually add more products to your routine to treat the various skin concerns you still want to address.**

Although there are products you may not want to use in the beginning, there are mandatory steps you must follow to take the best care of your skin, no matter what. **Proper, gentle cleansing, especially at night to remove makeup, is a must** because sleeping in makeup can lead to dull skin, breakouts, and red, puffy eyes. **Also a must is protecting skin every day with a sunscreen rated SPF 15 or greater. Another step, which will make a world of difference, is exfoliating on a regular basis with a well-formulated AHA or BHA:** You will see the difference after your first application. At night you must apply at least one product appropriate for your skin type that is loaded with antioxidants, skin-repairing ingredients, and cell-communicating ingredients. These are the product steps you should absolutely not skip!

DID YOU KNOW?

The four most essential skin-care products are:

1. A gentle cleanser
2. A daytime moisturizer with broad-spectrum sunscreen (SPF 15 or greater)
3. An AHA or BHA exfoliant
4. A moisturizer for dry areas and for use around the eyes

Visit *Beautypedia.com* for the top-rated products in all of these categories.

How can I tell if a product will make me break out?

> **"** Following are a few guidelines that will help you find the products that are least likely to cause blemishes:

In most respects, you cannot tell. Most of us who've struggled with breakouts have at one time or another used a product that claimed it wouldn't cause breakouts, yet we broke out while using it.

Why is it so tough to tell? Because it is hard to know which ingredients, and what concentration, will trigger breakouts—and this varies from person to person, so **the exact same products that make you break out may not make your friend or sister break out**, even if you have the same skin type or follow the same routine.

There's also the issue of concentration: Usually there's only a teeny amount of an ingredient in a skin-care product, which wouldn't be the same as a 100% concentration that might have been used in lab tests to determine whether or not the ingredient will cause breakouts. Plus, there are thousands of cosmetic ingredients to consider, many of which have never been subject to research to determine if they (or various combinations of them) will help breakouts, do nothing, or even make breakouts worse. The lists of ingredients to use or avoid based on their alleged ability to clog pores mean well but, in reality, aren't helpful.

What should you do? Following are a few guidelines that will help you find the products that are least likely to cause blemishes:

Avoid products with thick, overly creamy textures, or any products that come in stick form. The ingredients used to give a skin-care or makeup product a thick or solid texture are more likely to clog pores.

Products with a gel, light serum, liquid, or fluid lotion texture are far less likely to clog pores and cause breakouts.

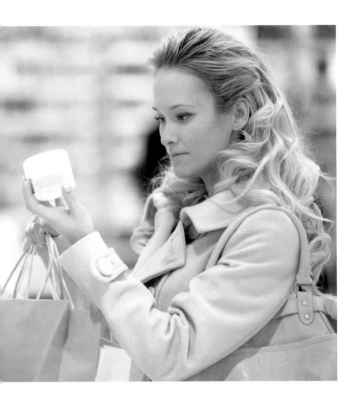

Oils of any kind do not actually clog pores, but they do make your skin feel greasy. That adds to the excess oil your skin already produces, thus exacerbating the conditions that lead to more blemishes.

Avoid products that contain any kind of irritant, such as alcohol, menthol, peppermint, eucalyptus, camphor, lemon, grapefruit, or lime as well as natural or synthetic fragrances. Irritation stimulates oil production at the base of the pore and that makes skin redder, makes red marks more noticeable, and hurts your skin's ability to heal.

When should I begin using anti-aging products?

As Paula often says, "From birth!" What she means is that there's no magic age when you should begin using anti-aging products, just as there isn't a specific age when you should start eating healthy, nutritious foods.

Remember—age is not a skin type! **Skin needs anti-aging ingredients throughout your lifetime and almost from birth it needs sun protection— you cannot begin too early; waiting to help your skin until you see wrinkles or other signs of sun damage or aging definitely doesn't make any sense.** So, whether you're 20 or 50, it's never too early to begin using anti-aging products. And it's 100% false that if you start "too early" the anti-aging products won't work when you really need them!

Ideally, anti-aging is about giving skin of any age more of what it needs to repair past damage, produce healthy collagen, and function properly so that it looks and feels healthier and acts more like younger skin. You'll find such products in our **Best Products section at** *Beautypedia.com*.

TO SUM IT UP:

Think of anti-aging skin care like a healthy diet: what's healthy for you to eat as a child will be just as nutritious throughout your life. It doesn't make sense to wait until you're unhealthy to begin eating healthy foods, and it doesn't make sense to wait to use anti-aging products until you see signs of aging. You cannot start too early, and doing so doesn't mean these products won't work when you really need them most!

How do I get rid of the stubborn dark circles around my eyes?

Buying yet another eye cream is not the answer for making dark circles around your eyes go away. Really—have any of them ever worked as claimed? Even the cosmetics companies don't believe their own claims about the eye creams they sell to lighten dark circles or reduce puffy eyes because if they did why would they launch new ones year after year after year, all making the same promises? If the previous ones worked as claimed, what are the new ones for?

Regardless of the exaggerated claims cosmetics companies make, there are definitely steps you can take to reduce dark circles. **Here's what you can do that will have the most impact:**

Because sun damage makes dark circles worse, always wear sunscreen around the eyes during the day. And, make sure it contains only zinc oxide and/or titanium dioxide as the active ingredients because they won't cause irritation, which can make dark circles worse.

Get more daily sun protection with sunglasses.

If you have allergies, consider talking to your physician about using an antihistamine. Allergies can be a major cause of dark circles.

At night, use an emollient moisturizer loaded with antioxidants around your eye area—and slather it on!

In the morning, apply a great concealer that is one or two shades lighter than your skin.

Remember, your under-eye moisturizer doesn't have to be labeled "eye cream." There is NO research showing that there are any special ingredients needed for the eye area. NONE! Brilliant ingredients for the face that fight dry skin, wrinkles and environmental damage and lighten dark areas and reduce inflammation work for the eye area, too.

What can I do about sagging skin and loss of firmness?

Many skin-care products claim they can firm, lift, and/or tighten sagging skin, but none of them really work to the extent claimed on the label or in the ads. **A face-lift-in-a-bottle isn't possible**—there are no skin-care products anywhere in the world that can come close to the results you get from medical procedures. **But, don't be discouraged. There is extensive research showing that if you use the right mix of products, you will see firmer skin that has a more lifted appearance**—you just need to be realistic about the results you expect to achieve. Here is what you need to know:

1. The elastin in skin is the reason it "bounces" back into place.

2. Young skin makes lots of elastin; older skin makes almost none.

3. Sun damage and age degrade elastin.

4. Research is clear that it is almost impossible for older skin to make more elastin, even with medical procedures.

5. Most firming creams are a ridiculous waste of money because they don't contain ingredients that can firm or tighten skin.

What works to firm and tighten skin? Although building more collagen doesn't help skin bounce back, it does help support skin, and you can help skin make lots of collagen by using skin-care products that contain potent antioxidants and skin-repairing ingredients.

Sunscreen is a must! Because sun damage destroys both elastin and collagen, daily sun protection is critical, but how many of us remember to apply sunscreen to our necks as well as our faces?

Using products that contain salicylic acid or glycolic acid really helps. While these ingredients are exfoliants, there is also a good amount of research showing they build more collagen and, to some extent, can firm skin.

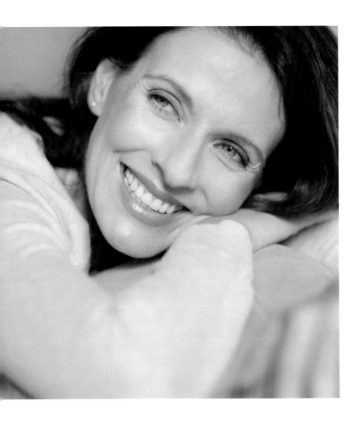

Retinol, applied topically, can definitely help your body build more collagen, and it can improve the shape of damaged elastin. There is a small amount of research showing that it can even help build new elastin.

Last, medical procedures such as lasers and other light therapies have impressive skin-firming results! Save the money you'd normally spend on expensive firming creams and facials, and soon you'll be able to afford these types of skin-changing treatments.

How do I reduce puffy eyes when nothing seems to work?

Put those cucumber slices and tea bags away because they aren't going to improve your puffy eyes. Here are some of the best things you can do to really help deflate puffy eyes:

- Sleep with your head slightly elevated to minimize fluid retention in the eye area.

- Reduce your alcohol and salt consumption; both can cause puffiness around the eyes.

- Keep your eyes well lubricated with artificial tear–type eyedrops, such as Allergan's Refresh brand.

- If you have allergies, ask your doctor about taking an antihistamine (such as Benadryl or Claritin) to reduce swelling.

- Avoid rubbing your eyes! Lots of people do this absentmindedly, so make sure you're aware, and then break the habit!

- Generously apply a moisturizer loaded with antioxidants to soothe and smooth skin around the eye area.

- Be sure to get all your makeup off every night! Sleeping in makeup is a sure way to cause puffy eyes.

- Never use skin-care or makeup products that contain irritants of any kind, including fragrance, around the eyes.

How often do I need to reapply my sunscreen during the day?

It depends on how much exposure to daylight you anticipate and how active you'll be while skin is exposed to daylight.

For casual wear, meaning less than four hours total time out in the sun, it is not necessary to reapply sunscreen rated SPF 15 or greater (and greater is better for continuous exposure to sun as opposed to intermittent exposure). If you are perspiring or spending a longer period of time outdoors, you should reapply your moisturizer with sunscreen.

Otherwise, the general guideline is: **Reapply sunscreen at least every two hours if you're outdoors and perspiring, and immediately after toweling off from a swim**, even if you're wearing a water-resistant sunscreen and weren't in the water too long.

What if your foundation is the product you've chosen for sun protection? Then the trick is to be sure you've applied it evenly and liberally. Pressed powder with sunscreen is a great way to add sun protection during the day. **A foundation and pressed powder with sunscreen are excellent options for those with oily or acne-prone skin** or for those who dislike the feel that's characteristic of many sunscreens—just be sure to apply a regular SPF product to your neck, arms, hands, and chest because they will be exposed to the sun, too. If you perspire heavily while wearing foundation with sunscreen, then you will need to reapply it to maintain sun protection.

> " Be sure to apply sunscreen to your neck, arms, hands, and chest because they will be exposed to the sun, too, and therefore age prematurely. "

What's the difference between serum and moisturizer? Do I need both?

Serums differ from moisturizers in two important ways. **First is texture:** Most serums typically are sheer, fluid-like, and often very silky, while moisturizers tend to have a gel, lotion, cream, or balm texture. **Second is purpose:** The chief function of serums, even those that contain moisturizing ingredients, is to deliver a concentrated dose of specialized ingredients (such as retinol or vitamin C) to skin. Moisturizers, on the other hand, are intended primarily to moisturize the skin, although if well formulated, they also should provide a concentrated dose of anti-aging and skin-repairing ingredients.

For best results, we advise using both–serums and moisturizers–applying either the serum or the moisturizer first. Those with oily skin may find that a serum provides all the moisture and healthy, essential ingredients their skin needs, although they may still need an emollient moisturizer for use around the eyes and on the neck.

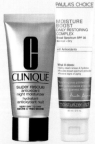

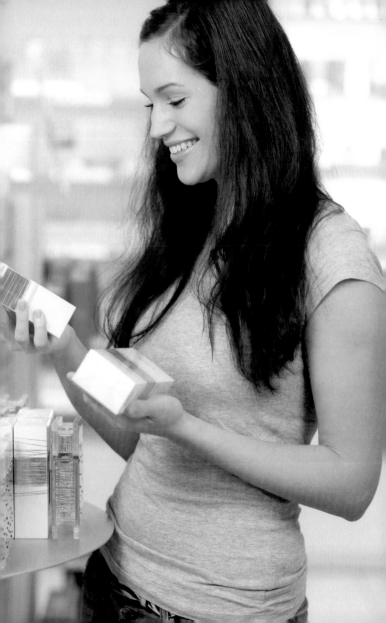

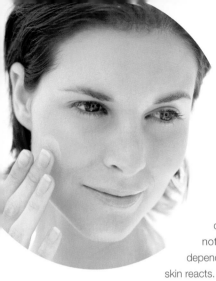

I have rosacea. Which anti-aging products can I use?

Many women with rosacea worry that their skin will react badly to anti-aging products because they tend to contain more "active" ingredients that can trigger a flare-up, but that's not always the case. It completely depends on the product and on how your skin reacts.

Rather than avoiding state-of-the-art anti-aging products altogether, look for those that don't contain fragrance (synthetic or natural), and don't use products that contain irritating plant extracts or oils. You absolutely should be using products that give skin an array of ingredients that can help rebuild its barrier function—a key factor in combating the symptoms of rosacea. Also, look for products that contain proven anti-inflammatory ingredients, as these help to calm skin and reduce redness.

Two more tips: Consider an AHA (containing glycolic or lactic acid) exfoliant carefully. A BHA (salicylic acid) exfoliant might be the best option because of its natural anti-inflammatory qualities, but be sure the BHA exfoliant contains other anti-irritants as well, and no irritating ingredients like alcohol.

For sunscreens, choose those with the gentle mineral active ingredients titanium dioxide and/or zinc oxide, as these are least likely to cause stinging or flare-ups.

To find the best products to use when you have rosacea, visit us at *Beautypedia.com*.

How do I handle dry skin and breakouts without making either worse?

Having breakouts, dry skin, and wrinkles at the same time is a common complaint for women—even if they didn't break out as teens. Given multiple issues like this, it can be confusing to decide which skin-care products you need. You really can address all of these issues at the same time if you use the right products, which is explained in the answer to the question about acne and wrinkles on the next page. The only difference? For the moisturizer step, use a richer moisturizer for dry areas not affected by breakouts and a lighter moisturizer on breakout-prone areas.

Which antioxidant is the best?

There isn't any one single miracle skin-care ingredient of any kind. Regardless of the story behind the ingredient, whether it is an exotic antioxidant like melons from the south of France or a rare flower or oil from the Amazon or Morocco, there simply isn't a best one for your skin. Instead, **there are dozens and dozens of effective antioxidants for skin,** ranging from familiar ones like green tea, grape extract, and vitamin C, to ones you may not be familiar with, such as idebenone, epigallocatechin-3-gallate, or superoxide dismutase. What counts is that the product you use contains a variety of these ingredients—and the more the better. **Research shows that skin does better with a cocktail of effective antioxidants rather than with just one.**

> " Research shows that skin does better with a cocktail of effective ingredients rather than with just one. "

I have acne and wrinkles, so how do I treat both?

Struggling with acne breakouts plus wrinkles can be frustrating and confusing. Here are the types of products you need to fight both at the same time:

1. **A gentle cleanser** that's water-soluble and contains soothing ingredients. No bar soaps or bar cleansers—both can be drying and the ingredients that keep bar soaps and cleansers in their bar form can clog pores.

2. **A BHA (salicylic acid) exfoliant to reduce breakouts, blackheads, white bumps, and wrinkles.** BHA also reduces red marks from past breakouts.

3. **A product containing benzoyl peroxide.** For more stubborn acne, add a gentle, fragrance-free product medicated with 2.5% or 5% benzoyl peroxide, the gold standard for killing acne-causing bacteria.

4. **A treatment serum loaded with anti-aging ingredients.** Most serums are lightweight, which makes them ideal for those with oily skin, breakouts, and wrinkles. The best ones are loaded with the antioxidants, skin-repairing substances, and cell-communicating ingredients all skin types need to look and act younger and healthier, and to help heal the red marks that blemishes often leave behind. These ingredients help repair signs of aging and stimulate collagen production, plus help skin heal and fight inflammation (a major component of acne). Talk about win-win!

5. **A lightweight, smoothing moisturizer.** Choose a moisturizer with either a very light, thin lotion feel or a gel texture loaded with antioxidants and skin-repairing ingredients. Your skin needs beneficial ingredients such as antioxidants to stimulate collagen production; anti-irritants to reduce both red marks and patches of dry, flaky skin; and softening ingredients to diminish the appearance of wrinkles. Apply at night after exfoliating and after applying your treatment serum.

6. **Daily sun protection.** Protecting your skin from further sun damage not only reduces and improves wrinkles, but helps combat breakouts, too! By preventing the inflammation that sun damage causes, you're

strengthening your skin, allowing its immune response to help heal breakouts faster! You need matte-finish sun protection from a product that smoothes and hydrates without making breakouts worse. You can also use a foundation and a powder with sunscreen as your daily facial sun protection. Make sure sunscreen application is the last step in your morning skin-care routine!

For specific product recommendations visit *Beautypedia.com*.

How do I get rid of red marks from past breakouts?

> **"** These ingredients help repair signs of aging and stimulate collagen production... **"**

Superficial red marks, which may be pink or brown depending on your skin color, can be so frustrating! Here's how to fade them faster:

Use only gentle skin-care products. Anything that irritates skin, such as harsh scrubs or products with alcohol or fragrant plant extracts, can worsen redness and impair healing.

Apply a well-formulated exfoliant containing salicylic acid. This step, done once or twice daily after cleansing and toning, can make a difference overnight!

Use a sunscreen rated SPF 15 or greater every day, no exceptions. Unprotected sun (daylight) exposure hurts your skin's ability to heal, even if you don't burn or tan.

Apply products loaded with antioxidants and skin-repairing ingredients. These ingredients are essential for helping reduce inflammation and allowing skin to heal.

For specific product recommendations visit *Beautypedia.com*.

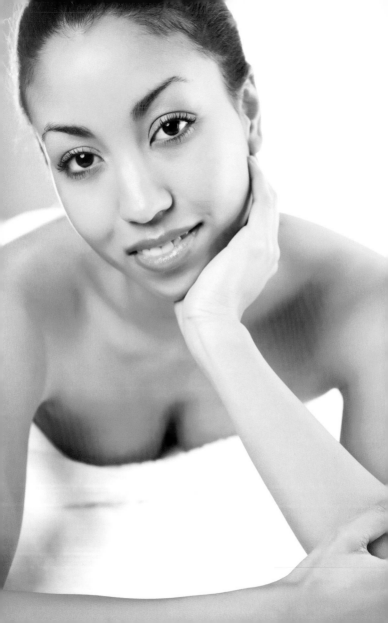

Should I use a prescription retinoid such as Renova and a skin-care product with retinol?

It isn't necessary to use both, but there's nothing wrong with doing so if that's your preference and if your skin responds favorably. Retinol in all its forms, over-the-counter or prescription, is excellent for preventing and improving signs of aging. But, for the over-the-counter version (i.e., cosmetic version), which contains the entire vitamin A/retinol molecule, to be effective, the molecule must be broken down into the active form (tretinoin), which is found in prescription vitamin A products. All of the retinol products we recommend are formulated to do just that.

Keep these facts in mind to help you determine which form is best for your needs:

- Prescription-strength forms of Vitamin A/retinol (tretinoin) are "stronger" and work faster. Cosmetic retinol takes longer to have an effect, but in the long run it works the same.

- Prescription-strength forms of vitamin A/retinol (tretinoin) present a greater risk of irritation, which may prevent ongoing use.

- Cosmetic retinol has a far lower risk of causing irritation, but because it is still breaking down in your skin to become the active prescription form (tretinoin), it also can be irritating.

- It takes experimenting to determine what frequency of application works best for you. Many find that using retinol 2–3 times per week works great, while others can use it every day.

If you decide to use a retinol product and a prescription retinoid, apply the retinol product in the morning and follow with sunscreen rated SPF 15 or greater. Apply the prescription retinoid product at night, followed by serum and/or moisturizer.

Is mineral makeup really special for skin (especially sensitive skin)?

No. In fact, mineral makeups are nothing more than loose or pressed powders with the word "mineral" on the label. They are not better for sensitive skin and they are not easier to use than other types of foundation. If anything, the loose types of mineral makeup can be extra messy!

Of course, some companies claim their mineral ingredients are the best, but there's no research proving that any mineral ingredient is better than any other. Plus, mineral makeups aren't any more "natural" than other products that are not labeled "mineral." In fact, most minerals must be synthetically treated to become cosmetically elegant.

Keep in mind that if you have dry skin, any powder can make it look drier, and if you have oily skin it can pool in pores. So, it's wise to use a magnifying mirror and check your makeup in good light to be sure you like the results.

If you're currently using mineral makeup and love the results, that's great, but it isn't any better for your skin or worth paying a lot of money for.

What are BB Creams and CC Creams? Do I need one?

BB and CC creams are popular all over the world because their does-it-all claims make them seem like miracles, but they aren't!

The term BB stands for either Beauty Balm or Blemish Balm; some companies call their versions CC for Color and Correct. It sounds new and it seems it might be a better way to multitask with one product, but that's not the case.

Regardless of the name, most BB and CC creams are little more than tinted moisturizers with or without sunscreen. Sometimes these products include beneficial ingredients, but sometimes they are poorly formulated, even lacking the ingredients necessary to provide reliable sun protection.

The fact is: Just because a product is labeled a BB cream or CC cream does not guarantee you're getting a superior "does-everything" product. For example, there are many tinted moisturizers with sunscreen that are not called BB or CC creams, but that work just as well or even better!

> "
> ...most BB and CC creams are little more than tinted moisturizers with or without sunscreen.
> "

YOU NEED TO KNOW:

- "BB" stands for "beauty balm" or "blemish balm"
- BB creams are essentially just tinted moisturizers
- It is the rare BB cream that contains an impressive amount of treatment ingredients
- The "does it all" claims for most BB creams apply to many foundations with sunscreen, too.

How do I choose the best foundation shade for me?

For most women, regardless of race or age, foundation should be some shade of neutral ivory, neutral beige, tan, dark brown, bronze brown, or ebony, without any orange, pink, rose, green, or blue (meaning an ashy/gray) undertones. In other words, think neutral colors!

Neutral shades work best for almost all skin tones. By "neutral," we mean shades without visible overtones of pink, peach, copper, ash, green, or yellow. Women with pink or ruddy skin or who have a natural red undertone or "green/ash" undertone, often choose foundations that match those shades. For women with lighter skin, their face ends up looking like a mask; for women with reddish skin tones, it enhances the red appearance, making skin look overly made up. On women with ashen undertones, choosing a foundation with this undertone can make skin look dull, as if it lacks radiance.

A neutral-tone foundation softens all skin tones and looks far more natural than trying to match pink, red, or ashen tones in your skin. However, regardless of our recommendations, always check your foundation choice in natural light so you know exactly what other people will be seeing.

Foundation should never "color" skin, rather it should be a smooth layer that evens out or enhances the skin tone and covers imperfections. You add color to your skin with blush and lipstick, not with foundation. In other words, foundation should be your secret, and not obvious to the rest of the world.

If I'm not sure which foundation shade is best, should I pick the lighter or darker color?

When in doubt about whether you should go lighter or darker, apply the foundation you are considering and compare the color at your hairline and neck (at the jawline) with the color on your face to be sure there is no glaring shade difference. This ensures a more natural appearance.

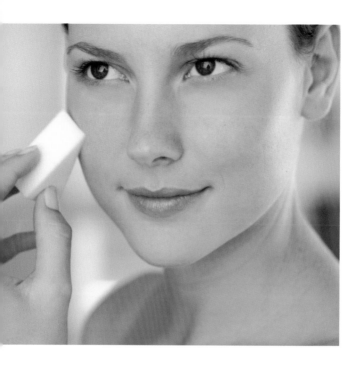

Most of the time, this means going with the lighter of the two shades between your neck and face, because if you choose the shade you think matches your face but not your neck, it will show an obvious line of demarcation where the two meet. Besides, you can always adjust a lighter foundation with powder and/or bronzing products; it's much more difficult to lighten a too-dark foundation and still look natural.

If your neck is a distinctly different color from your face, you should shop for a foundation that leans more toward matching your neck, or is somewhere in the middle, to minimize a mask-like foundation application. Whatever foundation you choose, be sure to check it in natural light so you know how it looks.

Visit *Beautypedia.com* for a list of the best foundations.

How do I determine my best shade of lipstick and lip gloss?

There's no firm rule to follow here, other than to make sure your blush and lip color are in the same color family. That means you should pair a rose-tone blush with a rose- or pink-tone lipstick. You shouldn't pair, for example, a peachy blush with a magenta lipstick because these colors clash and can make your face look harsh, which most women don't want.

You might have seen or heard recommendations that you should wear a shade of lipstick or gloss based on the color of your lips—that doesn't make any sense! The color of your lips has nothing to do with the shade of lip color you choose. Think about the colors you've seen on celebrities who look gorgeous—clearly these colors have nothing to do with their natural lip color.

A few ideas to consider when choosing shades of lipstick are as follows:

- Darker shades of lipstick can make lips look smaller and darken the appearance of the teeth.

- Very light or super-sheer lipsticks and glosses can make your skin look washed out and dull, especially at night.

- Don't be afraid to think outside the box and choose a color you haven't worn before, like red, fuchsia, or coral.

Also, there's no need to always match lipstick or gloss to your clothing, but if you're in the mood it can be fun to wear a red lipstick when you're wearing red or to go with the general color direction of your clothing. If the floral print you have on is more pink than coral, wear a shade of lipstick in that color family. You can consider matching your skin tone (warm or cool undertones), but that can end up clashing with your wardrobe depending on what you have on.

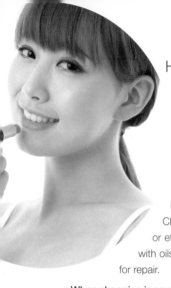

How do I solve the issue of dry, chapped lips?

The best thing you can do to treat and prevent chapped lips is to keep your lips covered with an emollient lip balm or gloss! You can restore dry lips with consistency and patience. Lip balms that are mostly wax (like the Chapstick brand) aren't nearly as helpful or effective as lip balms that blend waxes with oils, proven emollients, and antioxidants for repair.

When chapping is severe, or if you notice flaking along with a dry feeling, use a gentle lip scrub prior to applying the lip balm. The scrub quickly removes dead, dry, flaky skin and leaves a smooth surface for lip balm application. If you haven't tried a well-formulated lip scrub, prepare to be surprised at the results!

Watch out for lip products that contain skin irritants, such as menthol, camphor, peppermint, or citrus, or those that are highly fragranced. These ingredients have no benefit for the lips and end up compounding the problem. A classic example of this, and sold almost everywhere, is Carmex Lip Balm, which contains potent irritants that will have you reaching for more Carmex as your lips become drier, perhaps never realizing that it's the lip balm itself that's contributing to the problem.

> " If you haven't tried a well-formulated lip scrub, prepare to be surprised at the results! "

Which products are safe to use during pregnancy?

As a general rule, we recommend consulting your physician for advice on personal-care products used during pregnancy and/or if you plan to breastfeed your baby. However, most skin-care products, such as cleansers, toners, moisturizers, eye creams, scrubs, and lip balms that do not contain FDA-regulated over-the-counter ingredients are fine for use throughout your pregnancy.

Prescription and over-the-counter skin-care ingredients such as salicylic acid (BHA) are a different issue. Here's what you need to know to make informed decisions (based on information from the American College of Obstetricians and Gynecologists):

Hydroquinone, which is used to reduce dark spots, has not been tested on animals or humans in regard to its use during pregnancy, so there is no information to assess your risk. It is best to avoid using hydroquinone during pregnancy or while you are breastfeeding.

Benzoyl peroxide is an excellent ingredient to combat blemishes and is considered safe in low concentrations (5% or less) when you are pregnant.

Prescription topical antibiotics, such as erythromycin and clindamycin, are considered safe for use during pregnancy.

Salicylic acid (BHA) is a superior exfoliant for skin, but when used in high concentrations for professional peels, it is considered a risk when you are pregnant. However, the percentages in most skin-care products (2% or lower) are considered safe. You can consider using glycolic acid or lactic acid (AHA) exfoliants as an alternative during your pregnancy.

Sunscreen actives, as demonstrated in animal studies, are not known to be a risk during pregnancy. The American College of Obstetricians and Gynecologists has not found any of the alleged fears about sunscreen ingredients to be substantiated by medical research. Daily sunscreen use is strongly recommended by dermatologists.

Avoid **prescription retinoids** (e.g., Renova, Retin-A, Differin, Tazorac, and generic tretinoin) and over-the-counter products with retinol. If you normally use this type of product, consider switching to an anti-aging serum that does not contain retinol.

There is no documented concern about ingredients such as vitamin C, niacinamide, peptides, or other types of antioxidants and cell-communicating ingredients when used during pregnancy.

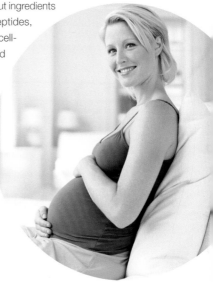

Ongoing use of skin-care products loaded with antioxidants and skin-repairing ingredients is highly recommended but, again, be sure to check with your physician and follow his or her advice.

We hope this guide has opened your eyes to the misinformation seen daily throughout much of the cosmetics industry. Paula and her team strive to bring you the truth behind cosmetics myths so you're kept informed and can make wise decisions about which products are right for your skin type and concerns. Along with our own Paula's Choice products and the products we recommend from other brands, the information in this guide reinforces our goal to help you take the best possible care of your skin!